INSTANT HYPNOSIS

the

EXPOSE

BY

Daryo Nagari

* * *

Copyright

Disclaimer

INTRODUCTION

Instant hypnosis is a fascinating subject for us all.

In the following pages you will get to know how they work why they work and how to use them. Before we start though a word of warning.

Some of the content describes how to relieve others of their possessions. These descriptions are for experimental and entertainment purposes only. If you choose to take part in criminal activities you only have yourself to blame.

This book is not intended as a training manual. The techniques described are for entertainment purposes only.

Any person using these techniques uses them at their own risk and discretion. You must always return any property taken during any prank you may choose to use.

It is not intended that you use these techniques to steal or otherwise interfere with or harm any persons.

Having said that Have fun. If you intend to go out and attempt these tricks my advice to you would be to record everything and have a written plan of action.

That way if you are questioned during the routine you can show that you are performing experiments and that you have no intention of robbing individuals or organizations.

PART ONE

Whether you have an interest in hypnosis or not you have probably seen a performance or two on the TV. You might have even been to a live performance either way you would have seen people acting out the most ridiculous things once they have been hypnotised.

If you have been to a live performance and seen this behavior, either by friends or family or even yourself.

You or someone you know may well have used a hypnotherapist to help with a phobia or undesirable habit.

Either way you will know that hypnosis exists.

Lots of people are interested in the phenomena. When I say phenomena I mean the things that happen once hypnotised.

Some of these sketches are brilliant.

Seeing a six foot tall alpha male dancing around a stage believing he is a female ballerina is priceless to his friends and family.

Watching someone eat an entire raw onion whilst experiencing eating a tasty apple is my favourite, even though it's an old one it certainly is timeless.

I have written this book not to talk about the phenomena or sketches but to talk about how to get someone to the state where they will perform them.

In hypnotherapy time is of no concern you book a one or two hour session and then you are carefully and calmly guided into a meditative state. Then you do some amazing realigning of your subconscious thinking patterns.

You leave therapy a rounder happier person.

When it comes to the entertainment side of things the hypnotist does not have the luxury of time. In fact he is up against the clock from the minute he appears on stage.

He needs to be hypnotizing people in seconds. After all once the volunteer or volunteers are up on stage his job is to entertain the other people left that is to say the audience. The audience has paid to be entertained after all.

And the volunteers have become the stars of the show.

Since the object of the show is to get the stars to perform and to be able to perform the stars have to be hypnotised it makes sense we need to do this rather rapidly.

The process of putting someone into hypnosis an induction because we are inducing the trance state.

On stage the hypnotist needs to use rapid and sometimes instant inductions. These are the impressive routines we have all seen which can sometimes give the appearance that a hypnotist has special powers.

For the record hypnotists do not have special powers, anyone can learn to hypnotise someone. Incidentally it's not that hard either.

The first thing to look at are some of the things you may have seen a stage hypnotist do when putting people into the trance.

On top of that there are the things that hypnotists do on the street.

The mind tricks

Handshake them into a trance

As a volunteer comes up onto the stage the hypnotist greets him or her.

Takes them to the centre of the stage and has a bit of banter with the audience and the volunteer.

He then says oh I forgot to introduce myself properly.

He brings his hand up for a handshake and so does the volunteer.

A few seconds later the volunteer's head is leaned forward the hypnotist is talking quietly to them about relaxation.

The volunteer was put into a trance just like that

The next thing you know the volunteer is performing.

First of all silly little things but after a while they are doing some seriously complex routines.

Such as the ballerina scenario mentioned previously.

Push them over into trance

Another either equally or even more impressive is when the volunteer arrives on stage, is brought to the centre or the stage.

The hypnotist again talks to him or her, the volunteer, and the audience.

While he is talking he is moving the star around quite a bit and showing them some little tricks to do with balance and standing.

Then in what seems like the blink of an eye the hypnotist pulls them backwards right down to the ground.

The volunteer is deeply hypnotised ready to take part in their own performance.

Once again they start with simple routines and gradually throughout the evening they are doing more and more complex things.

The wallet steal

This is not a regular stage show induction but is definitely worth a mention since it has been shown on television numerous times and looks astounding to those not in the know.

The hypnotist walks up to a guy in the street. Initiates a conversation and within a few seconds walks off with the victim's wallet and car keys.

As soon as the hypnotist disappears from view the victim visibly comes out of a daze and starts to realize he has just been robbed.

On TV the hypnotist returns the wallet and keys and explains to the victim he is on television etc.

Just for a moment imagine there were no cameras and the hypnotist was not performing as part of a prank!

You can see all over the internet news reports of people being robbed by hypnotists.

The victims always report that they handed over their belongings quite willingly.

Paid out for losing

Another street hypnosis 'trick' is the cashier hypnotised to give money to a customer for no apparent reason.

A famous television mentalist demonstrated this kind of instant hypnosis at a dog racing track in the UK.

He placed a bet for a race and the dog lost. He sent an assistant up to the claim window to confirm that the dog had indeed lost.

He then takes the same ticket back a few moments later to the same cashier and gets himself paid out as if he had won.

The cashier even confirms that mistakes cannot be rectified after he leaves. Then of course he leaves.

Click fingers

This is probably the most impressive of all inductions.

The volunteer is told to look at the hypnotist.

The hypnotist clicks his fingers and sends the volunteer into a deep hypnotic trance.

There are lots of variations of this.

The touching of the microphone to the head.

Touching the shoulder

In fact the possibilities are endless.

The important thing is that as soon as the hypnotist commands it the volunteer is asleep.

These are all examples rapid hypnosis being used.

In the following pages you will see how and why they work as well as how to do them yourself!

PART TWO

Hypnosis

The hypnotic trance is a state of mind somewhere between being awake and being asleep.

It's that point at night where you just drift off. Or in the morning as you wake up.

All a hypnotist does is recreates this state and then holds on to it for a longer period than usual.

Getting someone into hypnosis can be done in several ways

Relaxation

Focusing full attention

Shock

Confusion

A combination of two or more of the above is always best.

Traditional hypnotherapists use relaxation and

focus. They generally use the tried and tested method called Progressive Relaxation or 'PR'.

This method involves gradually relaxing the patient over an extended period whilst relaxing them gently down into hypnosis.

As mentioned earlier this is not the sort of thing hypnotists can use in the world of entertainment.

By the time they hypnotise a dozen or so volunteers they will end up with a group of hypnotized people on stage but the audience would have either fallen asleep through boredom or left altogether.

Good luck with his next show!

Hypnotists who work on stage use the other forms of induction Focus, shock and confusion. They use relaxation to deepen the hypnotic state but only spend a short time doing it.

They rely on the fact that each time a person follows a suggestion they become more suggestible. So effectively the show itself or at least the routines are the deepeners.

Deepeners are what they sound like a means of deepening the trance. The deeper a person is in trance the more suggestible they become.

Now we are going to break down the previously mentioned examples of the use of instant hypnosis.

Handshake

So first let's look at how the handshake induction is carried out in detail.

1/ The hypnotist brings his hand up in front of him as if to offer his hand for a greeting handshake.

This initiates a pattern. The volunteer then brings their own hand up to meet the hypnotists for a handshake.

This is part of our social makeup.

The important thing is that we don't have to think about it. We do it automatically. We do it unconsciously.

The unconscious takes over the handshake.

It expects the two hands to meet, for the fingers to close down in a grasping motion.

Then it expects that both arms will shake gently up and down together.

Then it expects to break contact.

This expected turn of events is quite rightly called a pattern.

We know this is done unconsciously because as we do it we continue with the verbal greeting and other niceties. And we cannot consciously do more than one thing.

2/ Right before the hands meet, the hypnotist takes the volunteers right wrist in his left hand and moves it up in front of his face.

This is called a pattern interrupt and if you have read the previous paragraph properly you will know why it is so called.

When you interrupt an unconscious pattern there is a moment of total shock and confusion.

It lasted for about a second.

It takes about a second for the unconscious to hand over control to the conscious.

The conscious mind is the reasoning mind. So you see the unconscious has had something unexpected happen and it is going to hand over to the conscious saying 'this didn't go according to plan you need to figure something out'

Fir the hypnotist the one second delay is all he needs.

During that second the mind as a whole is in complete limbo.

The unconscious is trying to gather itself. The conscious is not yet aware of any problem.

If left eventually after that all important

second it will make contact with the conscious and deliver its message

Then the shock and confusion will be over and the person will compensate.

In that second the hypnotist has a golden opportunity in that moment of absolute limbo the brain will accept anything in the interest of feeling OK.

So the soothing voice of the hypnotist is like a tonic and is accepted without challenge.

3/ the hypnotist brings the hand up in front of the volunteers face. This limits the amount of external visual inputs.

what the hypnotist says during this time is not that critical. As I mentioned above the mind wants anything as long as it's something.

The most popular thing to say is of course sleep, but you could say armadillo if you wanted. As long as within that one second you say something.

What is critical is that you continue talking because now that you have spoken the unconscious has accepted you as the safe voice. The hypnotist's voice saved them from limbo.

This means that the voice is in charge. And so the hypnotist is now in charge.

If the hypnotist says nothing the volunteer will come out of his trance in a few seconds. That transition of the power from unconscious to conscious will sort of 'kick in' gradually if left to its own devices.

This is because of two phenomena Fast in Fast out. And fast in deeply under.

So once you have saved the unconscious with your initial word of comfort the hypnotist needs to keep talking and directing. This will keep them in deep trance quite easily.

4/ Obviously the hypnotist can say anything to keep the volunteer just as they are, on the edge of the limbo state, Ideally he needs to guide them into a deeper hypnotic state, the deeper the volunteer goes the more easily he will carry out the suggestions given him during the 'show'

Once the hand is in front of the face the hypnotist has two choices.

Choice number one is to tell the volunteer to stare at their hand and concentrate on all the features thereof.

Tell them to take note of every single detail.

Then move on after a minute or so to deepening by suggesting more relaxation or deeper trance.

So this method would be using pattern interrupt combined with narrowing attention followed by deepening.

Choice two the hypnotist puts the hand up to

the volunteer's forehead and commands sleep. Then pulls the hand, along with the head, down whilst encouraging depth of trance and depth of relaxation.

This would be a pattern interrupt followed directly by a deepener by a deepener

The pull down.

1/ the hypnotist approaches the volunteer and physically moves them around by the shoulders gently but firmly.

Changing their position and aspect on the stage.

He may say to the volunteer face left.

Then as they move around to their left the hypnotist just moves them along.

Since the hypnotist is putting on a show he will engage the audience and return to the volunteer at intervals.

Each time he returns he will reposition the volunteer by telling them where to stand etc and follow that instruction up with the physical 'helping'.

When done properly it seems like nothing untoward is happening, or at worst the hypnotist can't quite make up his mind where he wants his volunteer to stand.

This could not be further from the truth.

This moving around and getting the volunteer to obey little commands is a vital part of the routine.

By doing this the hypnotist is sending a strong and subtle message to the volunteers unconscious.

Every time the volunteer complies with both

the verbal and physical encouragement he is being programmed to obey.

2/ the hypnotist then holds on to the volunteer and taps his feet together.

This is again a forceful compliance maneuver.

It also has the added effect of making the volunteer slightly unstable. Since with the feet together, the centre of gravity is closer to the edge of the base.

The base of course is the volunteers the feet.

3/ next the hypnotist moves the person around by the shoulders encouraging them to let go and trust the hypnotist not to let him (the volunteer) to fall over.

This movement back and forth side to side etc increases the instability of the volunteer.

Also when the hypnotist moves the volunteer around he tells them what he is doing.

So if he pulls them back slightly he accompanies the physical movement with verbal conditioning such as. As I move you backwards just let yourself go, backwards where I tell you.

Then he will continue by pulling the volunteer forward saying that's right allow your whole body to move forward because I won't let you fall.

This again is very powerful conditioning, what is happening for the unconscious is this.

It is obeying the commands to allow his body to go where he is told to let it go, continuing the compliance.

The unconscious though has no understanding of time, to it things just 'are'. So we end up with a chicken and egg situation.

Did the hypnotist move me then tell me to move or did I move because he told me to. It doesn't bother trying to figure it out, it just accepts that whet the hypnotist says happens

4/ now the hypnotist is ready, he stands in such a way as to catch the volunteer.

Or he has a helper with him.

He stands behind the volunteer and to the side, usually facing the audience.

He then reaches around the volunteer places his hand on the volunteer's forehead and pulls back.

The volunteer falls backwards of course.

As he passes through the point of no return, which is not far since his feet are together the hypnotist commands sleep.

The volunteer is lowered all the way down to the ground.

They were in a hypnotic trance about halfway from vertical to horizontal by the way.

So what has happened here is we have gained compliance by ordering the volunteer around. In turn the volunteer has put the hypnotist in control. When the hypnotist does the pull back the volunteer experiences a shock. Similar to the pattern interrupt only this time it is pure shock.

It is the feeling we all have had if you ever swung on a chair at school.

Sometimes you go too far and in that second before you fall or grab a table and pull yourself back, the unconscious is handing over control to the conscious.

If you remember that feeling of 'blind' terror then you know the feeling.

A better phrase would be blank terror because the mind cannot process anything except 'HELP'

Once again as the mind cries for help the friendly hypnotist is on hand to offer assistance. This time in the form of a loud command to sleep. And the volunteer happily complies.

So in summary we have had.

Conditioning and shock.

The wallet steal

This is a kind of instant waking hypnosis

If you look back to the handshake induction I said there that fast in is deeply under.

This is the part of the phenomena we use to take the wallet, keys or whatever. The downside is that fast in is fast out.

That is why on film the victim comes around in a few seconds after being 'mugged' and comes in search of the hypnotist.

1/ the hypnotist approaches someone in the street, he holds something in his hands a can of drink or similar. He asks directions in a positive frame.

This is to say that he suggests where he wants to go is in a certain direction at the same time he points in that direction.

The victim also points the hypnotist raises his arm so that it exactly mirrors the arm of the victim.

The victim agrees that the hypnotist is indeed right in his assumption that the place he is looking for is in the direction they are both pointing.

The hypnotist then repeats the statement one or even two times, varying the language, something like so up that way is where I want to go?

Again the victim agrees and point. The hypnotist points too.

What happens here is that the hypnotist is doing two things. He is getting the victim to agree with him, by using yes statements. Remember the subconscious does not recognize time.

So it is already becoming a little confused about who is leading the conversation.

By getting the victim to keep saying yes he is agreeing to agree subliminally to everything the hypnotist suggests.

The other thing that is happening is the hypnotist is disarming the victim and making him feel safe and off guard.

This is done by raising the arm and facing the victim at the same angle as the victim is standing.

So if his legs are pointing at ten to two across his body then so does the hypnotists.

This is called matching. We feel comfortable around people we perceive as the same as us. When the hypnotist matches the victim with his body language he is saying ' we are the same, you are completely safe with yourself/ me'

Once he has matched the victim the hypnotist starts to lead.

So first the hypnotist raised his arm after the victim then he raises his arm before. He goes from matching to leading. In the NLP world this is called pacing.

You can mirror match and pace in other ways too. A very effective but subtle one is breating.

That's the purpose of the repeated statements. It gives him a chance to put his arm up and reposition his body, when the victim follows suit he is just about ready to move in for the 'kill'

2/the hypnotist brings his hand up for a handshake as he says thanks for that. Thanks for giving me that. As the victim brings his hand up for the handshake the hypnotist once again points in the direction of the location he is looking for.

You can see what has happened. The pattern interrupt is initiated, remember when you interrupt that pattern the unconscious is screaming to be rescued and given guidance or instruction. The instruction that was given is. 'Giving me'

The victim is now in an eyes open hypnotic trance.

3/the hypnotist then offers his can of drink for the victim to hold on to. At the same time telling the victim to give him his wallet.

The victim happily places the wallet in the hypnotist's hand, and then the hypnotist continues with confusing the victim by taking back his drink and handing the victim back his wallet and then the drink telling him to hold onto those for me.

Then the hypnotist says OK thanks that, or give me those, repeating one of the patterns set up earlier in the routine.

He points at the wallet. Again the victim hands

over the wallet.

The hypnotist takes his can of drink back. He thanks the victim for his help and leaves.

His final command to the victim is 'you were walking that' way and points him in the opposite direction.

The victim walks away. A few seconds later the victim visibly stunned starts to come out of the trance and comes to find the hypnotist. All is revealed to him secret cameras, everything.

So let's have a look at the entire routine in brief to see what happened.

The hypnotist gets compliance through the yes statements.

He mirrors the victim.

He then begins to lead.

Then he uses a modified pattern interrupt

And continues to talk to sooth the subconscious

As well as keeping the victim confused.

Then he simply commands the victim to hand over his goods and chatels.

Of course at the end the victim is made aware that he is now a TV star and is given his wallet back.

The scary thing about this use of hypnosis is

that an unscrupulous person could use this routine to steal for real.

I am not going to tell you how since this would be irresponsible, and to be quite frank you've probably worked it out anyway.

I would say that only ever use this for fun and make sure you return the belongings!

The dog track

Or the Jedi mind trick

The dog track routine again as seen on TV can just as easily be done at a horse race track too. It is not so easily done in the UK since bets and payout references are made by the name of the horse not the number under which it is running. In the USA though, bets etc are made against the number of the horse.

1/ the hypnotist places a bet on a dog it doesn't matter what number it is. However some numbers are more useful than others when it comes to the covert verbal instructions.

If the dog wins fine pick up your winnings. If it loses well…Go and pick up your winnings!

2/ the hypnotist goes up to the payout window and presents the ticket to the attendant. The attendant checks the ticket and passes it back to the hypnotist. Telling him it's not the winner.

So far there has been no subterfuge.

3/ the hypnotist does not take the ticket back instead he looks her straight in the eye with a hypnotic stare.

This makes her feel uncomfortable. No doubt in the past she has had hardened gamblers very upset at her window upset and angry, maybe even violent.

This creates an air of expectancy that something may happen. This phenomenon is discussed later. But because her unconscious is expecting something, even though she has no idea what, there is an element of preconditioning.

4/ before she has time to become too alarmed he says could you check it again.

Now the attendant takes the ticket again.

At this point she is just going through the motions of checking to keep the customer happy.

Perfect for the hypnotist, this is a key moment.

As she takes the ticket a second time she is about to run through a mind numbing routine that she does hundreds of times a day. A subconscious pattern, exactly as mentioned earlier.

5/ the hypnotist slams his hand on the window and in an authoritative tone says.

'This is the dog you are looking for'.

She continues checking the ticket and after a few seconds pays out on the losing ticket as if it is a winner.

She pays out because the mundane routine pattern of checking a ticket was interrupted.

Yes our old friend the pattern interrupt.

In this case though it is not so easy because there is no handshake and the attendant is not participating on a personal level. in fact she is about three feet away.

Let's look at the language used and the inflections.

So firstly he uses an authoritative tone.

This puts the employee in her place unconsciously.

The phrase ' this is the dog you are looking for' the unconscious subliminal message is the dogs number.

Since four was indeed the winning dog, and he says the words 'IS and LOOK and for in a different tone to the rest of the sentence. As well as elongating the words very slightly.

She hears 'this **IS** the dog you are **look**ing **four**'.

So this emphasizes the words 'is, look and four' and at the same time makes it a command word.

When your voice deepens at the end of a sentence it makes the sentence a command, if you go to the extreme it turns into a threat.

By elongating slightly too gives it more meaning than the rest of the sentence.

To prove a point to the man accompanying him, the hypnotist did this 'trick' again.

When he went to a second window he did exactly the same with an added and powerful subliminal command to reinforce the claim.

He did the same slamming of the window and the command to pay out, but added something to seal the deal.

Whilst the second attendant was checking the ticket he told her 'that's why we came to this window.

Again same voice tonality and he says the word window in two parts splitting the syllables. Win-dow. Implying that it is a **WIN**dow.

I also call this the Jedi mind trick routine since it sounds just like the line from the movie star wars.

'These are not the droids you're looking for.'

Because of the remoteness of the attendant this is not a routine for the feint hearted, you need all the help you can get. The fact that the winning dog number is four helps the hypnotist cause.

You can say it no matter what dog wins. But you could also hedge your bets by modifying the sentence slightly.

You could say this is the one you are looking for. Becomes this is the WON you are looking for. If the number one dog did win that's an added bonus.

Click and sleep

The most impressive of all instant inductions.

The hypnotist walks up to the volunteer and clicks his fingers in front of their face and commands sleep! The volunteer duly falls straight into a deep trance.

Most of the time this is a false representation. The click/ sleep is usually a re-induction.

That is to say that the volunteer is already hypnotised or has been hypnotised and the hypnotist is putting them back under.

Most people do not realize this but when you watch a stage show although the volunteers appear to be woken and put back in trance several times during the performance this is not really what is happening.

The people on stage stay in trance for the entire show. The hypnotist simply takes them from eyes closed trance to eyes open trance and back again.

The fingers clicking are set up as a trigger. And when the trigger is 'fired' as we say. The volunteer shuts their eyes. No different than any of the other skits.

When you hear this music you will dance like a ballerina. Etc.

Take nothing away from the click sleep trigger. It looks dramatic to the audience and is an evergreen favourite.

There is another added bonus to the click/ sleep phenomena.

That is that each time the volunteer closes their eyes to the sleep command they become more deeply hypnotised. And of course, more suggestible.

There is an exception to this rule that click and sleep is only a re-induction and that will be discussed later in the book.

PART THREE

summary

A word about how to identify who to try to use instant inductions on.

Regardless of the kind of hypnosis being used it is common practice to carry out what are known as suggestibility exercises.

These are tests carried out by volunteers in order to gauge how easily they can be hypnotised and how suggestible they will be.

There are very many exercises but they all relate to the same thing.

The hypnotist is looking for people:

Who have a good level of concentration; remember we want to be able to narrow their focus to the exclusion of all outside stimulus.

Who can follow instructions without question?

And most importantly have an excellent imagination.

As I say these are standard tests or exercises to determine the suitability of the hypnotist's volunteers.

I have a slightly different view on this.

Since I know that everyone is hypnotizable. That everyone gets better at being hypnotised with training I am of the opinion that the objective of the exercises is not to see who the best potential subject is.

I think that the tests and any following show content should be used to create good hypnotic subjects.

There are a lot of hypnosis comedy acts out there some good some not so.

The tried and tested method for performers is to get a dozen or so volunteers on stage more if there is room, then do suggestibility tests.

Once they've done these tests they put everyone into a light trance. Then they proceed to whittle down the volunteers into the 'best' hypnotics.

By this I mean that the volunteers who did well in the tests get used more and the ones who did less well do not get used at all.

It is not unusual to see a hypnotist on stage with twenty volunteers using only two or three to do the more difficult routines.

If the hypnotist were to use the tests and the skits/ sketches to bring the 'weaker' subjects along he could end up with twenty people on stage all doing difficult routines. This is impressive stuff.

Hypnotists who do these stage shows according to the 'hypnosis stage performers manual' (doesn't exist by the way) *that's my attempt at sarcasm*, are missing an opportunity and could be doing themselves a great disservice.

If the hypnotist does the first suggestibility test, sees his good candidates and rearranges the stage so that the weaker ones are in the centre of the stage with the stronger ones to their outsides they are more easily influenced by the others. And they improve.

They are influenced because they see others under the power of the hypnotist and they start to believe and indeed expect it to happen to them.

Another advantage is that when the instantly inductions start the weaker ones become more and more convinced that something will happen. Create expectation and they will believe that something will happen and then it does.

If enough expectancy and belief is created during the initial induction there comes a point when the click and sleep exception I mentioned earlier becomes a reality.

If someone watches the hypnotist perform instant inductions on half a dozen or so other volunteers they are so in awe and expectant that the hypnotist can often walk straight up to them click his fingers and say sleep and they are gone.

Tests

Before we look at a couple of exercises I should mention that they are impractical for the covert street stuff like the wallet steal and the Jedi mind trick.

So two tests that are good to use to start a show.

The hypnotist has the volunteers stand in a semi circle so they can see him and each other.

They are instructed to hold their hands up in front of them prayer style with their hands grasped together.

They are told to use their.

Intelligence

Imagination

Concentration

And to do exactly as they are told.

They are told to imagine their hands are stuck together.

Really imagine it. Then they are told that each time the hypnotist touches their hand they are to imagine that the hands are ten times more stuck.

The hypnotist then goes around and around touching the hands of the volunteers and repeating the suggestions.

After a couple of minutes once the hypnotist is happy they are all really trying.

He tells them that they can try to unstuck their hands but the harder they try to separate them the harder it will be to separate them.

Anyone who does not succeed with this is dismissed. That should only be a couple if any.

The hypnotist should then release them from this spell

Another good exercise

The volunteers hold their hands up in front of them at shoulder height about eighteen inches apart.

The hypnotists suggest the hands are magnetically being pulled towards each other.

These suggestions are repeated until everyone's hands are moving towards each other.

The added bonus with these magnetized hands is that when volunteers hands get close to each other.

The hypnotist can go to them push their hands together and shock them into trance. It is a really smooth transition. And once again it helps to convince anyone who is struggling a bit.

Now You Know

So now you know how it all works.

Watching a hypnotist perform will never be the same again.

You now know that before he even asks for volunteers he is creating an atmosphere of awe. Which helped with the audience's expectation?

Then he gives the safety advice this is not only a legal requirement but it does sow a small seed of fear into the audience.

You know exactly why he has as many volunteers as possible and why he gets them to clench their fists.

Most importantly you now know how he sends his volunteers into a deep trance in second's right before your eyes.

So you see that as he hypnotizes one person after the next he creates more belief and expectation in others.

With enough people on stage he may even get to the point where he can use the click/ sleep routine cold!

Well that's all folks I hope you enjoy and remember.

Use responsibly!

Thank you

If you have enjoyed reading this book please tell others.

Also I would appreciate it very much if you would go to the site from which you purchased it and left some feedback for me.

My other books all available at Amazon are

Speed hypnosis for therapy

Body language exposed

Waking Self Hypnosis

Join the Dots

Stories that Heal

Thanks again

Daryo Nagari

Copyright